Cover photography by: Casey Cottrill
Editing by: Elaine Abel

ISBN 9781689985406 (Paperback)

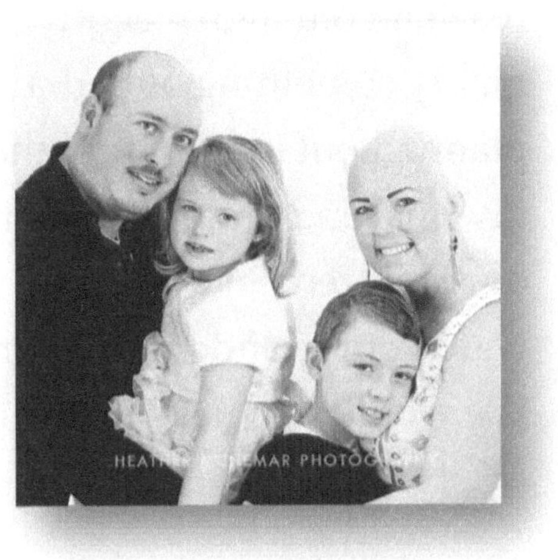

Introduction

Life doesn't always turn out
how we imagined. We have
this perfect picture in our head
of how it should be. If you're
like me, sometimes you think
you're invincible and your
health will be fine until you

reach an old age of eighty or ninety something. I had it planned out in my mind that my husband and I would raise our children, and one day watch our grandchildren grow. We would live happily ever after.

At such a young age I never imagined that I would ever be faced head-on with cancer. That my life would be turned upside down. That "perfectly planned-out life", it would be something completely different. I felt like it was the end of life. Honestly, I looked at it as if I was Mario, in a video game and when my diagnosis came, I thought to myself *"game over!"*. I laugh at that now, but that's really, how it felt.

My family, friends and community were so wonderful to pick me up when I fell. I had tremendous support throughout the most difficult time of my life. From the many calls, messages, cards and company, I could feel the love from all.

One day, soon after my diagnosis, I had lunch with Mary-Helen, a friend from church. She told me about her battle with breast cancer years before and we discussed my upcoming treatments. She might not know it, but that time with her was a turning point for me. She lifted my spirits and gave me hope that day!

I began reaching out to others near my hometown that had been or were going through their own battle with cancer. Facebook had several support groups, so I joined a few and was surprised to find so many women within a few counties of me that were fighting breast cancer, and some a few states away. They were all different ages and some just weeks ahead of me in treatment.

I began chatting with these women every day, sometimes a couple of times a day. We held each other up and created a bond that could never be broken. Whenever a "pink sister" was hurt, we would all hurt. If someone was newly diagnosed, we welcomed them with open arms. When a sister lost her courageous battle, we would mourn together like she was one of our closest friends. More than anything, we gave each other HOPE.

Having cancer taught me many things in this beautiful life, one of them being empathy. The meaning of empathy is: *the ability to understand and share the feelings of another.* I think after going through times of difficulty, you begin to understand what others are feeling. Before I went through this trial, I could try to imagine the pain others were feeling, but it really didn't measure up to what they felt. During my own battle, I made a promise to God that I would be a light for others through their fight.

My prayer is that this book falls into the hands of someone who could use a little hope in their lives. Whether you've been diagnosed with cancer or are facing a difficult season in life, I pass on my courageous story of faith, hope and love.

<u>Chapter 1</u>

*"For the battle is not yours, but
God's."*

2 Chronicles 20:15

"God's got this!" I said to my gynecologist as I was leaving her office that beautiful, warm day, September 15, 2015. I was filled with confidence as I left and headed to the hospital for an ultrasound. My doctor had just discovered a lump in my left breast.

When I arrived at the hospital, they took me back to change into a gown and had me lay on the table. A little bit of fear crept in. My heart started beating a little harder. This lump looked scary. Could it be cancer? I was only thirty-three years old and I had two young children. This couldn't be it. The harder the xray tech pushed on my breast with that wand, the more painful it became. I wished that someone could have been there with me, but as usual, I felt like I had a handle on things and jumped into it myself. After the tech finished up, she left the room so I could change. I noticed she left an image up on the screen, so I took a quick photo with my phone and texted it to my sister-in-law before leaving. She was an ultrasound tech and I figured maybe she could help ease my fears. She also showed it to a few of her tech friends, but texted later and said they were not really sure. Even if she did know, I'm glad that she didn't tell me. Looking back, it probably would have had me googling breast cancer and scaring the heebie jeebies out of myself even more. So, thank you, Brandi!

That week, we had a rummage sale at our church and I volunteered to help. I figured it would keep my mind on other things so, I worked that morning with my Grandma and a sweet friend, Sonnie. My grandma was asking me questions about the ultrasound and when I might hear back from my doctor. I had not told anyone but a few friends and family, so Sonnie asked if she could pray with us. I

was all for the prayers at that point! I really think it's a beautiful thing when someone prays for you. It shows how much they really care. After the prayer and a few hugs, our pastor walked in. He talked a few minutes and then I pulled him aside, told him what was going on and asked if I could

be added to the prayer list. Of
course, he said yes, and then he
said, "Let's not worry too much
about it until there's something
to worry about." My Pastor is
an easy- going fella that loves
life and has an incredible faith
in God. No worries with this
guy. He can tell you, if you ask
him exactly how many days he
has been on this earth. He's
very inspiring! He went to his
office and grabbed a book and
told me that I needed to read it.
The book is titled "20,000 Days
and Counting" by Robert D.
Smith. In the book it teaches
you to be intentional with your
life and to live in the moment.
So, in this moment, as I'm
writing this book, I have been

on this earth for 13,706 days. Wow! I hope

that I live for another 13,706 days. I guarantee that if I get to, then I'll live it with more purpose.

Two days went by and I was at my mother-inlaw's playing with the kids when my phone rang. It was my gynecologist with the results of my ultrasound. She said "We received the results and it is a solid mass. You will need to be set up with a surgeon." She recommended a great facility, Betty Puskar Breast Care Center. In that moment, I actually felt at peace, knowing that, 1) God has this! and 2)

They'll just remove it in surgery and all will be well! In my mind I thought- *"There's no way I have cancer. That's crazy!, I have nothing to worry about!"*.

My doctor transferred all of my files to the breast care facility, and they had me set early the next week for a biopsy. I tired to take it easy that weekend and relax with my family at home. No better medicine for the soul than that.

A few days quickly passed and we were headed to my appointment. My step-mom, Denise came with us. She was great company, that would help ease both mine and my husband's minds, especially since we didn't know what to expect.

We arrived at the breast care facility, I checked in and we sat down. The nurse was pretty quick to call me back, but she told us that my husband and step-mom could not come back with me. She took me back and showed me to a dressing room and lockers. It reminded me of a store dressing room and the lockers reminded me of school. It was very calming, the lighting was lowered and I believe there was music playing. I changed into a pretty pink gown, put my belongings into the locker and stepped out into the hall. The nurse took me

to another waiting room, where
I would wait to see the doctor.
It was a calming atmosphere as
well, there was a tv playing,
some magazines on a coffee
table. Instead of chairs they had
couches; I guess you could say
it felt like home. What didn't
feel too much like home were
the other women sitting around
the room in pink gowns. I think
they were all playing it cool, as
was I. I gazed around the room
and looked at each one,
wondering if they were as
nervous as I was. About ten
minutes after sitting there, a
nurse called out my name. I
thought- *Here we go, let's just get
this over with!* I followed her
back to a room and was greeted

by two other nurses. They were all very nice and made me feel comfortable. One nurse prepped me while the ultrasound tech turned on her machine. They gave me four shots of lidocaine to numb my breast and the doctor made her way into the room. She introduced herself and began getting all of the instruments in order that she would be using. She explained to me that while the tech had the ultrasound wand over my breast, she would then insert the needle into the mass. It was actually pretty cool to watch. The mass looked similar to a kidney bean and the needle just pulled cells from within. After she collected from the mass, she implanted a breast marker, which is used to identify the area where breast tissue is removed. She indicated that on my previous ultrasound, something looked fishy under my armpit. So, she also took a needle biopsy of a lymph node. My body started shaking, I wasn't sure if it was my nerves, but I just couldn't lay still. She finished pretty quickly and as she left the room one of the nurses asked if they needed to take me for a mammogram. Her reply "No, I have what I need." Ummm, I'm questioning in my head-

Is that bad? Does she know that it doesn't look good? Maybe it's good, maybe it just looks like a cyst and she's confident. The nurses sat me up and I instantly felt very nauseas and couldn't quit shaking. They brought me some crackers and juice then mentioned that was why they ask you to eat right before arriving for your appointment. These were the side effects of lidocaine. While I was having a little snack, the nurses stood around me asking what I did for a living and whether I had any children. I can't say enough good about that place. The atmosphere and the staff knew exactly how to make you feel like you didn't have this burden or health scare looming over your head. After I finished, they sent me back to the changing room. I was relieved it was over with and couldn't wait to get on the road so I could see my kids. In this whirlwind of an emotional week, God and my family were keeping me sane.

<u>Chapter 2</u>

"Be still and know that I am God."

Psalm 46:10

In my normal day-to-day I was busy running a photography business. It was plenty to keep my mind occupied. For once in my adulthood I felt like I had accomplished so much and was in a good place, doing what I loved every day. On the inside though, my health was taking a toll. I was working a full-time job at a car dealership while also trying to get my photography business off of the ground. My biological mother whom I had an off and on relationship with was dying. I was also trying to keep up with my kids, husband, and everyday life.

Growing up, my Dad was single, taking care of my brother Wayne, sister Elizabeth and I. I'm sure it was hard. He was working a fulltime job and keeping up with us. My grandma helped-out a lot and we also had great sitters. One of my favorite parts about childhood was that my Dad took us to the beach every year. Still today, I feel like if I don't visit the beach each summer, then have I truly lived? Haha!

We started attending Christian Fellowship Church about my kindergarten year of school. I remember the day Pastor Ed stopped by and invited us to church (which we still attend today). We were eating pb&j sandwiches with mac-n-cheese and running around like crazy kids. Ah, memories. I was too little to understand, but him stopping by and giving that invitation was a turning point for us, all for the better.

When I was about eight or nine years old my Dad married my Step-Mom, Denise and we gained two sisters, Rachel and Sarah. Sometimes life with the brady bunch was crazy and hectic. It wasn't too long before all of us kids fought like actual brothers and sisters. Today, we still do, especially in our group text messages. I'm the calm one though, that sits back and watches it all unfold. While eating popcorn. Sometimes I'll turn it on night mode when I've heard enough. But, in all seriousness, we wouldn't trade it for the world. We love each other like blood and would go to the ends of the earth for each other.

We continued attending CFC throughout the years and I look back now and see all of the blessings that God has brought into our lives. Here you have my dad, who was raising three young children on his own, he fell in love a few years later and we gained two more siblings. I'm sure our parent's prayers have gotten us through some pretty tough spots in our lives. I guess I didn't even realize that they prayed until I saw my dad knelt down beside his bed with hands folded and eyes closed. I knew not to bother him, so I just kept on walking, but how special to see that. I hope my kids see Jesus in me as I have seen in my parents.

We each are now grown with families of our own. My parents are grandparents of twelve happy, healthy grandchildren! That's pretty amazing right there. For my parents to have the great love that they do, and to have an abundance of blessings. What more do we need in this life than each other?

I married my husband James about a year after graduating high school. Five years later we had our first baby, Nathan. He brought so much joy to our lives. Three years later we brought our beautiful daughter, Catie into the world. I began working at the car dealership when Catie was about eight months old. I also had my first dslr camera and took so many pictures of the kids. I would post them on social media and the photography took off from there. I loved both jobs. Although I had grown in my job at the dealership, my ultimate dream was to have the photography business flourish having it as my only fulltime job. I worked so hard at trying to make that dream a reality.

In February 2015, all my dreams came crashing down as I experienced the worst anxiety I had ever felt. It was so bad that I couldn't even leave my house and go to work. I felt like a prisoner inside of my own body. I knew that most of the anxiety had come from trying to be everything to everyone and chasing after dreams that were too far out of reach. Looking back, I'm sure hormones and an imbalance of something in my body made up the rest.

One morning I woke up about five o'clock and felt like I couldn't breathe. My mind was going about a hundred miles an hour and I was shaking. It was, simply awful. I was on a medicine daily for anxiety, and also had a prescription of Ativan for emergency uses. Generally, the Ativan helped within fifteen minutes of taking it, but I remember laying there that morning and thinking,

I didn't actually have thoughts of suicide, but at that moment, I didn't want to be here on this earth any longer. I felt like a complete failure as a mother, wife, daughter, employee.

Just a let-down to everyone to be honest. I hated how my body felt day in and day out.

I stumbled out of bed, took an Ativan and then sat down on the couch. I picked up my phone and logged onto Facebook to try and occupy my mind until the medicine kicked in. As soon as my newsfeed refreshed, the first post I saw was from a church friend. She wrote "Be still and know that I am God". I don't know what clicked in my brain, but as soon as I read that verse, I thought to myself- "Why had I not turned my troubles over to God? He is all I need!" I started sobbing and talking to God. I said "God, please help me, come into my life, I give everything to you. Please forgive me of all of my sins, Lord I give you my life!" As I sat there praying, this peace, the kind of peace that surpasses all understanding, came over my body.

No, no, it wasn't the Ativan. It had not been in my body long enough. I knew that this was a different kind of peace. There is no medicine that had ever made me feel like this before. This peace came from God. It was the kind that I heard about at church, in stories, on tv. I felt like a new person! Still today, when I think about that moment, I have chill bumps all over and when I talk about it, I still choke up and start crying. I love to tell the story. If you know me, I'm sure you've heard it. If you know me and have not heard it until now, I would be happy to share it with you!

After talking to God that morning, I showered and got the kids up and ready for school. I played hooky from work that day and needed to thank my church friend, Robin. I stopped at the flower shop, picked up a beautiful bouquet and a card. I filled the card with my story of what had happened that morning after seeing her post on Facebook, and I thanked her. I dropped the flowers off at the school she taught at and stopped over to visit my grandma since she just lived a few minutes from there. I had to tell someone what had happened that morning and seeing that my beautiful grandma was one of the first ones that I told anything to, it was perfect!

Later that day in the afternoon I received a message from Robin. She wanted to thank me for the flowers and said that she typed the bible verse out that morning, but erased it, then God told her to type it back out and post it. Isn't that amazing? God works in mysterious ways! From that day on, Robin has been one of my best friends.

 As the day went on, I still felt great! I cleaned the house up, the kids came home from school, we worked on homework and then I started dinner. I told my husband what had happened as we sat down to eat dinner. About half-way through eating I just felt very tired, and a little sick to my stomach, so I excused myself from the table and laid down on the couch. It was all very weird. I'm sure my husband was thinking, "What in the world?". That was a little after six in the evening and I fell into a deep sleep. I didn't hear them cleaning up from dinner and didn't even hear everyone go to bed.

I woke up about eleven that night to the sound of my phone ringing. By the time I got myself together I noticed it was a missed call from my Aunt Sue. I also noticed I had several missed messages from the past couple of hours.

I glanced at the first message saying something along the lines that my mother had been taken to the hospital and was unresponsive and that they had been trying to revive her. I was getting ready to call my aunt back, when another aunt had texted and said, "she is gone." My heart sank, my mind raced. I immediately felt like I couldn't breathe, and I went straight for an Ativan before a fullblown panic attack came on. It was like I had forgotten all about the peace God had blanketed me with that morning and tried to handle it on my own.

I woke my husband up to tell him the news and he sat and hugged me until I fell asleep. The next few days were spent with family and in those quiet moments I sat and thought about how bad that day would have ended if God had not showed up that morning and turned my life around. Soon after my mother's passing, I quit my job at the dealership, and I took the plunge to try the photography business full-time. My husband and I talked about it and decided if this would make me happy then let's do it! Life is short! How very true when we hear – God is always on time! It blows me away thinking about it today, five years later.

Chapter 3

Trying to take it easy since my biopsy just two days before, I had decided to take a drive to town and pick up some craft show fliers for a friend. I had them printed at a local print shop on the college campus in our hometown, where my Step-Mom works. She's located in another building from where I was heading, but occasionally when I'm by there, I'll pop in and say hello. That afternoon though I needed to pick the fliers up and head back to the school to pick up the kids. Catie had dance and then Nathan had soccer that evening.

 I headed into the building and pushed the elevator button to go up a few floors. For some odd reason the elevator was taking its good ol' time. As I was patiently waiting, my phone started ringing. Above the number calling it said 'Morgantown, WV'. My heart started racing; it had to be the results from my biopsy. I answered and nobody was there. The reception must have been poor in the building, so I ran outside, but they had hung up by the time I made it out. With shaky hands I tried holding my phone still while calling the number back. A lady answered and I told her who I was. She stated that she had just called me. Then what she said next felt like a punch to the stomach. She said, "*The results of your biopsy show that you do have breast cancer.*" I dropped to my knees. This couldn't be real. I was only thirty-three years old. I had two young kids. They needed their Mother. As all of these things were going through my head, she was rattling off the type of breast cancer I had and telling me that I already had a team of doctors ready to meet me the following week. I could barely keep it together as I found a pen, but my hand was shaking so bad that I couldn't hardly hold it.

She told me that I had Stage II Invasive Ductal Carcinoma breast cancer and gave me the name of my oncologist along with the date of my appointment.

After finishing the call, I picked myself up off the ground. I tried to compose myself the best that I could as I went back into the building. As I was

paying for my print service
upstairs, my hands and voice
were shaky as can be. It took
everything in me to not break
down. I made my way back
downstairs and out the front of
the building. I needed to tell
someone. My husband was at
work. I could have called him,
but my Step-Mom was closer. I
texted her and asked if she
would meet me outside, that
the doctor had called, and it
wasn't good news.

I started walking to her
building and saw her coming
towards me. I think we both
ran and embraced as soon as
we met. I burst out crying and
told her it was cancer. She held

me while I sobbed. Even though it was a very sad moment, it was a beautiful moment to me. I felt a bond there that I had craved my whole life from my biological Mother. I had never felt that with my Step-Mom. I think it was one of those 'God' moments. He knows exactly what we need, when we need it. I felt a little better after crying it out. She told me to not worry myself and to not search it on Google! Oh, she knows me all too well!

As I was heading up the road to get the kids from school my husband was leaving work and called me. I, of course burst out into tears again and told him the news. He tried to settle me down over the phone so I could drive. We decided to call our neighbor to pick our daughter up and take her to dance class right after school, while my husband said he would pick up our son and take him to soccer practice. The kids couldn't see me like this. I wasn't ready to deliver this awful news to them. Anything to protect them and keep some normalcy for as long as we could.

I remember sitting on the porch swing that evening while everyone was gone. I cried more and more, asking God to please be with me. I never imagined having to go through something like this. It was all so new, scary and felt overwhelming at the time. I knew God didn't make this happen to me, but it was a test of true faith. It was only a little over a year that I dedicated my life to Him. I remember a few months before my diagnosis that I was a little confused and wondered what my calling in this life was. I would pray over and over asking God to show me the way in which I should go. I was a Mom, wife and photographer, but I felt that there was much so more that he wanted to show me. I would say *"Here I am Lord, send me!"*. I've heard the saying before,

"Be careful what you pray for". I just didn't think this is where that would go.

While sitting there I texted a few friends to tell them. My parents told all of my siblings and I asked if they could tell my grandma. I knew if I told her personally, that nothing would come out. I would cry more than anything. My sister Rachel called, and I almost didn't answer her because I knew I couldn't talk. I said hello and that was it, we both cried until we hung up.

The next morning, I felt so at peace. I knew Jesus was with me, already doing what He had promised. Rachel texted and said she was stopping over, so I went out on the porch until she arrived. I met her at the end of the sidewalk, she hugged me tight and cried. To my surprise I didn't cry, and she joked about how she was a mess and I was more calm than she was. She handed me a package and inside was a breast cancer awareness shirt, pink nail polish and a pink headband (Insert heart emoji).

The next few days I received so much love from family, friends and the community. To be starting on the toughest journey in my life, it lifted my spirits and felt great to have so many in my corner.

<u>Chapter 4</u>

God is in the midst of her;

she shall not be moved.

God will help her when morning dawns.

Psalm 46:5

About a week after my results were in and it was indeed breast cancer, we again headed to Morgantown to meet with my team of doctors. My lovely Step-Mom took the trip with us as we would need an extra listening ear. I'm sure I was of no help that day. I was still in shock and my body was numb from the news. I felt like I was in a bubble and life was passing me by in slow motion.

We arrived at the cancer center, checked in and had a seat in the waiting room. I looked around the room, looking at the many patients that I would probably be hanging out with over the next couple of months. After a few minutes my name was called, and we were taken to a room. My first appointment that morning was to meet my oncologist, Dr Mehmi. Instantly my stomach was in knots. I knew as soon as he came in to see me that this journey was official. It was like a bad dream that I just wanted to wake up from.

Dr Mehmi was new at the center. He had moved from Florida where he practiced at a cancer center and upon meeting him, made me feel right at home here. We only spoke about what he knew from my biopsy about the type of cancer my mass was, the size, etc. He said that I would be having a PET scan and MRI the next week at the hospital and said we would know more after that. The PET scan would determine if I had cancer anywhere else in my body and the MRI would show more in-depth photos of the mass. Once he finished, we saw my surgeon, Dr Partin. I loved the way she carried herself. Very confident in what she was doing, and very personable. She gave us so much information about what we might expect with surgery and we went through my family history. I had bloodwork while there to send off for genetic testing. Although there is no history of breast cancer in my family, they wanted to make sure I didn't carry the gene, in which case my siblings or children might need to be further tested.

With all of this information we headed home for the day, after a long and tiring morning. As we were leaving, we talked about how great the doctors were that would be taking care of me. It was pretty quiet the rest of the way home, which gave me time to think. Think quietly to myself. I hated that I was going to be such a burden to my family. They would be running me up to the cancer center just about every week for the next few months. I cried under my dark sunglasses. I cried for my family, especially my kids. Why did they have to go through this? Why, why why??

The kids still didn't know about my cancer, but I knew I had to tell them soon, especially before I began chemo. I wasn't sure what to expect and if I ended up sick, they would ask a lot of questions. Every time in those last few weeks that I would try to find the right opportunity to tell them, I would go into panic mode. My palms would be sweaty, I would start shaking and felt like I couldn't breathe.

When they arrived home from school one evening that week, we were all sitting in the living room talking about our day. Thinking about how I could start the conversation and explain it in a way that wouldn't scare them. I asked Nathan if he thought he could cook dinner sometime. He replied with *"I know how to make grilled cheese."* We all chuckled, and I said *"You might have to help your Dad with dinner the next couple months. Mommy is sick and the medicine I'll be taking might make me sleep a lot."* They were both very quiet and I continued to tell them that I had cancer and I would lose my hair from the chemo treatments. It was a little awkward as we all just sat there. Nathan stared out the window while Catie asked a few questions. It didn't surprise me any though. Nathan is the one who worries about everything and Catie lets things roll off her shoulder. As we continued to talk, even about other things from our day, Nathan wouldn't look at us, as if he was in a trance. I knew he was pondering the news we just broke to him. He was eight years old, but I just wanted to scoop him up into my arms and make everything better. Eventually as the evening went on and we went outside to play, he seemed in a better mood, but I knew deep down that my news was really bothering him.

Later that week the port was placed under the skin in my chest, opposite of the mass. The port is a device made of plastic that has a small flexible tube that is guided into a large vein above the right side of the heart. A needle is inserted through the skin into the port to either draw blood or to give chemo. So much easier than using veins in your arm. The type of chemo I was administered would blow a vein. Yikes! The good thing about this surgery, is that I was able to go home afterwards. No hospital stay.

That weekend my mother's family traveled in from North Carolina. We had a nice visit and I loved the family time, but still, the freshness of the diagnosis had me in a depressed mood. My aunt surprised me with a pillow made out of a breast cancer awareness shirt that my Mom had. What if this was the last time that I saw them? When I had my health, it was easy to hear or say those words *"Just cherish the moment"*, *"Cherish the small things"*. But until you are faced with death, those words are raw. You feel them deep down, with every feeling inside of you.

After the weekend, we headed back to the cancer center for another appointment with my oncologist, bloodwork, PET scan and MRI. Dr Mehmi discussed my bloodwork and sent me off for scans. Sometime over the weekend I had developed a cold that felt like it was traveling to my chest, so it was a little hard laying still for the PET scan. I remember coughing so hard the whole thirty minutes that I had to lay there. They kept telling me to stay as still as I could, but it was almost impossible. Afterwards they took me down the hall for an MRI. Thank goodness it was so much easier and only took about fifteen minutes.

The very next morning I received a call from my oncologist. I trembled a little while answering the phone and was prepared to hear the worst possible news. He said, "*Hi Shanda, we received the results from the scans, and it looks like you have a little bit of pneumonia.*" I think I said something along the lines of, "*That's it? So, just the one mass? No other cancer?*" He replied with "*Just the one mass, no other cancer.*" He also told me that I would be starting chemo immediately. In fact, that Friday. He said that the results from the MRI showed that my cancer was ER/PR positive, HER2 negative and my mass was now 3.6cm. I had gone from stage 2 to 3. The tumor was growing fast. He called in a strong antibiotic to the pharmacy immediately so I could kick the pneumonia. I had four days to start feeling better before beginning chemo.

Thursday came and I didn't feel much better, so I headed to my local doctor's office. She gave me a shot of prednisone and some cough medicine. I was very worried that I wouldn't get any better by morning and that the chemo would make me very sick. My fear was hospitalization and trying to fight the pneumonia along with chemotherapy in my body.

As I did every day, multiple times a day, I asked God that night to help my body prepare for what it would be going through. I was comforted in knowing that even through my tears of worry, He was one step ahead, already making a way, just like He always does.

Chapter 5

*So do not fear, for I am
with you;*

*Do not be dismayed,
for I am your God.*

*I will strengthen you
and help you;*

I will uphold you

with my righteous right hand.

Isaiah 41:10

I woke up the morning of
chemo feeling like a million

bucks! That shot the day before really helped, but most importantly I knew that God had me in the palm of his hand.

We had to be there early that morning about 7:30, so that meant we needed to leave our house around 5:30am. I wasn't a fan.

On the trip up to the cancer center I was told to put lidocaine cream on my port site and then cover it with the small plastic wrap that was provided about 30 minutes before arriving. Once we arrived, I checked in and we took a seat.

The waiting room wasn't too busy at first, but after awhile, it started to fill. Again, I sat there in amazement at how many were there to be seen. These patients ranged in age from their twenties, all the way up to eighties and nineties. I like to study people, I wanted to know what their stories were, and I wanted them all to survive this horrible disease. As I was lost in studying these people, my name was called. A helper was waiting for me across the waiting room. Once I made it over to her, she put my bracelet on and told my husband that he would have to take a seat until we were finished with my labs. She took me on back to a smaller waiting room. I noticed while sitting in the chair that there was a pretty big window across the room from me. It was early in the morning and the sun had just risen over the parking lot out front. It was a beautiful sight. The warm sun beams came through the window and covered me. It was one of those God-moments where I sat in awe. It would be one of those few minutes that I would have to talk with God and set my mind straight right before having chemo each week. After about ten minutes a nurse called my name and walked me into another room with a curtain and I took a seat. She brought in several things and set on the little table beside me. She then wiped the lidocaine off of my port site.

Once it was dry, she took a little needle and inserted it into the port. I was pretty numb, so I didn't feel too much. She proceeded to take blood from it so they could send to the lab. There they would check potassium, calcium, bilirubin, magnesium, bun, chloride and several other levels. This would basically tell them if it was ok to do chemo.

The nurse kept the iv in my port, taped the small cords to my chest and then she called my husband from the waiting room. A guy met us in the hallway and took us to our room to wait on my doctor. Once there, our nurse, Laryann came to greet us. She asked how I was doing, and she sat there, truly listening, not rushing us. I knew we were in the right place. I told her I was ready to fight this and move on. I had to be positive and believe that God was already ahead of me. I knew that was the only way I would make it through this.

After talking to my nurse, Dr Mehmi came in. He went over bloodwork with us and asked how I was feeling. Most of it is a blur, but I'm sure I told him something along the lines of *"Let's do this!"*. We headed up to the next floor where the infusion room was located.

Again, we checked in and took
a seat in the waiting room.
Anytime my husband is
nervous, he picks on me. That
morning there was a lot of
picking. Generally, I would tell
him to stop, but I needed to
laugh, it calmed my nerves
some. I was admiring the bell
on the wall by the door. I
thought to myself, wow, five
months of chemo seems like a
very long time. I tried to
imagine what it would be like
to ring that bell. With no clue
what I was getting into,
I was stepping into faith. Faith
in God, that He would walk me
through the hardest situation
I've ever faced in my life.
Things were about to get so

real. I would lean on Jesus more than I ever had before.

A nurse called out my name. She took us around the infusion room, showing us where the nurse's station was as we went by. I'm just guessing, but I would say for every five infusion chairs there was a nurse's station. The chairs sat back in their own little room that held another chair and a television. There was a curtain across the door for privacy.

I took a seat in the big infusion chair. The nurse went back to her station to gather some fluids and meds, then back to our room to scan my bracelet and meds to put into the computer system. She then hooked up the iv meds to my port and explained that before each chemo I would have "pre-meds". The first meds were anti-nausea, acid reflux and steroids, which only took less than thirty seconds to give. Next came the fun part. I had really only had Ativan in a pill form or a shot in the rear. She gave the Ativan slowly through the iv, it worked so fast and relaxed me like no other. My husband made a comment that I probably didn't need my phone after taking it. Haha! I believe I did post a selfie on Facebook.

By that time, I was starting to get very hungry, so the nurse brought me a juice and some pretzels. She told us that the pre-meds had to work for about 30-45 minutes before chemo would be started. The type of chemo I was having was Adriamycin and Cytoxin. Adriamycin aka "red devil" was red, like Kool-Aid. It took about twenty minutes and was given through the port as well. When the nurse administers this, she puts on a full gown, mask and gloves. She had to manually push it through my port from a syringe. While she was pushing it through, I had to eat a popsicle, so I didn't get blisters in my mouth. Once that was done, she hooked up the Cytoxin. It's clear, like a bag of fluids and took about 45 minutes. After we finished up the nurse put a little sticky patch on my arm called Neulasta. It had a timer that would beep the next afternoon and give me an injection. This was given to promote white blood cell production. I would say, all in all, we were there for about 2 hours.

The ride home was pretty quiet, thanks to the Ativan. So, I slipped on my sunglasses and napped the whole way back. A few hours after returning home it was time for the kids to get out of school. By then I had a pretty good nap and the steroids were good at keeping me awake the next day or so. I felt pretty good the morning after chemo, but by the evening, a few hours after the Neulasta injection, I was very tired. I started taking some anti-nausea meds, and Claritin for the bone pain. The next few days after were tough. It felt like I had the flu. I remember laying back on the couch, trying to stay awake while the kids ran in and out of the house playing and hanging out with their Dad. I was fighting the sleep, but it wasn't long before I said to myself- *just rest, take a nap, let your body heal.* As long as I kept up on my meds for about four days after chemo, then every day I started feeling more like myself.

I was scheduled to take four rounds of this "red devil" combo every two weeks. By the time I felt like myself, it was time for another round.

Chapter 6

<u>Waiting Times</u>

*Waiting times are
growing times and
learning times.*

*As you quiet your
heart, you enter His
peace…*

*as you sense your
weakness, you receive
His strength…*

*as you lay down your
will, you hear His
calling.*

*When you mount up,
you are being lifted by
the wind of His
spirit…*

*when you move ahead,
you are sensitive to
His timing…*

*when you act, you
joyfully give yourself*

*to the things He has
asked you to do.*

-Roy Lessin

*Rest in the Lord and
wait patiently for
Him. -Psalm 37:7*

Halloween came about a month into chemo. I'm not a huge fan of this holiday but will celebrate with the kids. I love to see what they imagine up in their little heads and want to dress up as each year and do the traditional stops at Grandparents houses before going trick or treating. That year was a bit different.
I had chemo about two days before Halloween night. Normally I would be sleeping, a lot. I felt like I couldn't miss this moment though. We took the kids to their Grandparents for a bit,

where I was able to sit in a
chair and rest. From there we
drove to town and parked in
our usual spot, but I was too
weak to get out and walk. I sat
in the car while my husband
took the kids up the street,
door to door. It might not seem
like a big deal to some, but it
was so sad, I watched until I
saw them round the corner to
head up the next street and I
sat there and bawled. It was the
time with them that I wanted
the most, to make those
memories that we do every
year. But cancer took that from
me. You better believe that I
soaked up every second after
we made it back home. We sat
in the floor and sorted candy.

Nathan gave Catie all of his chocolate if she gave him all of her gum. It was the usual candy sort, just like every year and my heart was content.

There are other moments that blow you away or completely warm your heart. Like how Nathan's soccer team went out of their way to make me feel special. We were headed to a game one evening, and after pulling in at the field he took his ball and water, ran off to the field and as he was running away from the truck I noticed he had on a pink t-shirt and had thrown his jersey in the back seat. Once we made it over to the field, I noticed other little boys running in pink shirts. Even the coach wore pink! They played a great game and afterwards surprised me with a poster decorated that read "Team Shanda" and they huddled with me to take a picture. My son still has that poster hanging in his room, four years later. (Insert heart emoji here!)

I can't say enough about the wonderful community around us. I had friends send flowers, baked goods, so many heartfelt cards, texts, Facebook messages, phone calls, and the list goes on! My friend Natalie organized meals to be delivered the first four to five days after each chemo. It all just meant so much. I was blessed to have that support when I needed it most. I also had become friends on Facebook with a few ladies that were going through their own breast cancer journeys. Talking to them made me feel like I wasn't alone. They were dealing with the same side effects and feelings as I was. On days that I wasn't feeling myself, I would start chatting with them and suddenly everything was better. It did wonders for me! Reach out if you know someone that has been through what you're going through or vice versa. Don't be afraid to tell your story! If through telling my story, it helps one person, then I've done my job.

I can remember getting up the morning of my second chemo treatment and I just dreaded it. I laid there in bed and asked the Lord to give me the strength I needed to get through the day. I was like a cat, when someone is trying to give it a bath and it's clawing on for dear life not wanting to get in. Yep, that was me, leaving my house that day. I just didn't wanna! But on the drive up to the cancer center I received a text from my friend Robin. She was a school teacher and had my nephew in her class. She sent a picture of him with pink in his hair. The text read:

This precious little guy couldn't wait to tell me that he had pink hair for his Aunt Shanda. I asked him if he knew how much I loved his Aunt Shanda, he answered and said my mommy told me. Then gave me a big Roman smile and said I love her too.

Lifting you in prayer and already know that God has you cradled in His loving and healing arms. Remember- you are a daughter of the King!

God is always there for us and in some of the most unexpected ways! Later after arriving at the hospital, having bloodwork and meeting with my oncologist, he told me that the results of my MRI a few weeks before had shown some spots on my other breast that needed to be further checked out. So, they sent me next door to the breast care center for an ultrasound. Once in there it was determined that the three spots on my other breast were benign. That was a huge sigh of relief, but my oncologist had reassured that even if they showed malignant, the chemo would get them. While we were in ultrasound, the nurse decided to take a look at my cancerous tumor to see if it had changed in size. To our surprise it had shrunk, nearly in half! This was only after one chemo treatment. I had also used frankincense oil over the tumor site a few times after a friend suggested that it would shrink tumors. By that point, I was ready to try anything. I truly believe that God was playing an even bigger role in this than the medicine though. I felt his presence from the very beginning. This was an aggressive type cancer, but my God was one step ahead of it.

Around the second treatment, my scalp started to be so sore.

The ache all over my head was awful, it was almost like a nagging toothache. That weekend the kids were staying at my parent's house and we skipped church Sunday morning. These treatments wore me out and I only left the bed to go straight to the couch. My husband and I watched tv for awhile then he decided to take a quick shower before the kids arrived. While he was gone the pain on my head continued to intensify. It helped some when I massaged the back of my head, so after doing that a few minutes I pulled my hand away and pulled out a huge clump of hair. It was like a punch to the gut and so devastating! If you knew me, you knew I was always into my hair. I colored it at least every six weeks, tried out new hairstyles, it was never the same. So, to have my hair fall out, it was like the end of the world. By the time my husband came back into the living room, I was sitting there gripping onto the clump of hair and sobbing. He called hair salons to see who could get me in on a Sunday with no luck. I got ahold of my sister, Rachel and her mother in law, Pam took us in that afternoon. We called my parents on the way and asked them to keep the kids awhile longer. My sister sat in a chair across from me, while my husband stood at the doorway. As soon as Pam started cutting my hair off the tears started streaming down my face. I looked over and Rachel was crying too. My husband told us to both stop crying before he started himself. I was so angry. I thought *How dare this cancer!? It's only been a few weeks and its already taking pieces of me!*

Later in the day the kids arrived home. It was an adjustment for them to see me without hair. Nathan asked that evening if I was going to go put a wig on. I could tell it was really going to bother him. Catie on the other hand was wearing my wigs and dancing around the house. My momma bear-protectiveness was coming out and I really didn't want to see him hurt. It was one of the firsts that would break my heart during this journey.

Just like everything that had been thrown my way those last few weeks, I picked myself up, and tried to find the positive in the bad. It was very hard and a little embarrassing to not have hair. The wigs were very itchy, so I wore hats more often. One evening we met some family for dinner and after arriving there it was a little warm in the restaurant, so I took my hat off.

I had dressed a little nice and put some dangle earrings on that evening. I walked up to the salad bar to help my daughter and before heading back to my seat a gentleman walked up to me, put his arm around my shoulder and said *"I don't know you, but I just wanted to tell you how beautiful you are."* That guy doesn't know what he did for me. My confidence grew so much that evening!

A few days after my fourth and final "red devil" treatment we were getting ready for my sons ninth birthday party. We had invited all of our family and several of his friends. When we were getting ready to head out the door, I asked my husband if I should wear a hat or wig. I didn't mind going anywhere without, but there were going to be several kids and I didn't want to scare one of them. Nathan must have heard our conversation because he peeked his head around the corner and said "*Just go bald, don't wear a wig.*" It took me by surprise, but I went without as he suggested, and I don't remember getting any weird looks from his friends. I was so worried that Nathan might be embarrassed, but to have him tell me that I was okay without, it meant so much to me. (Insert all the heart emojis)

Chapter 7

*"Come to Me, all who are weary
and heavily burdened, and I will
give you rest."*

Matthew 11:28

About a week after my son's
party, I started on my first
Taxol treatment. This time
instead of every two weeks, I
had to go once every week for

twelve weeks. The doctor said the hard part was over and these weekly treatments would be easier. They were definitely easier, but whew, with each treatment I grew so much more tired than ever before. There wasn't but one or two days that I started feeling like my old self before it was time for the next one.

One of the worst parts about these treatments were having to take so many steroids. I would not only have to take them as my pre-meds on chemo day, but the night before I had to take five of them after dinner. I didn't like anything about them! They were good for something and that was to keep me from having an allergic reaction. I know first-hand too because I forgot them one evening. So, after that chemo I broke out in a horrible rash. It wasn't one bit fun, and it lingered towards the end of the rest of treatments. Speaking of pre-meds, instead of Ativan for this chemo, they infused Benadryl through my port after the steroids. The first treatment totally scared my husband. The nurse sent the Benadryl through a little too fast and they said my head hit the pillow instantly and I was asleep. He said he thought something happened to me. So, she said that she would put in my notes that I need it taken slowly. Most of the time the

Benadryl would still knock me out, but just for half hour or so and I would wake up long enough to talk to the nurse as she hooked up the chemo to my port. One morning, in particular she came in with her paper gown on and hooking everything up, I looked at her and said "I love that dress! It's so pretty!" Haha! I thought my husband was going to fall off of his chair cackling. I can only imagine all of the things the nurses have heard after the effects of Benadryl! We have to find the humor in bad situations like this, right?!

My fourth Taxol treatment fell on December 23, the day before my birthday. I was feeling well enough and wanted to show my appreciation to the nurses, so I took in several boxes of baked goodies. I wasn't sure about taking one to my oncologist because he seemed like a spinach and kale guy, but his nurse said *"Are you kidding? We have to hide our snacks, or he'll eat them all!"* We had a good chuckle out of that one. We took several boxes up to the infusion floor. There were so many great nurses that took care of me. I think they were pretty appreciative of the chocolate covered pretzels and peanut butter balls. In fact, I think the boxes were empty by the time my chemo was finished that morning. It honestly felt so good to do something for them, as they do so much for so many others, every single day.

We celebrated my birthday the next day. I felt ok, just a little tired. The kids were excited for me to open some gifts, but ultimately, I just wanted them close to me, it was all I needed. It's funny to think back before my cancer diagnosis, when I loved receiving gifts. I certainly wasn't greedy, but human. When I was younger my parents and grandparents would ask me to write birthday/Christmas lists. Still as I'm older, they, including my husband will ask. It used to be *Oooh! Anything that I want?* Now, I'm happy as can be if it's a kitchen towel or new underwear!

But really, all I really want is my family near. That's what I absolutely love about Christmas. We're so lucky to celebrate with both of our families on that day. We'll start by visiting my in-laws first for a few hours, then head to my parents. We save my family for later as the kids love to hang out with their cousins in the afternoon. We can usually plan it where all of us kids and our own kids are there together. It's very crowded, but we wouldn't want it any other way.

We spent a couple hours at my parent's house and then the noise from all of us crowded together started to bother me. I couldn't focus to talk to anybody, and I was exhausted. I usually don't want to leave until everyone else heads home, but to have to leave and go home early because I was sick, it really stunk. I gave hugs to all of my family and began to cry. The holidays really got to me. For one I hated that this disease took that precious time from us, and secondly, half-way through treatments, I still had a fear that the cancer would spread, and my life would end. So, each day, each holiday, each birthday is a gift from God, and I thank Him for that.

Chapter 8

It's so amazing to see the
human body at work. That first
week in January I spotted a few
hairs on my head. My hair was
starting to grow back! This was
a great thing to see! It created a
fresh, new feeling inside of me.
It was a great way to start the
year and finish fighting this
cancer. I had a new perspective

on life, and I couldn't wait to see where God would take me.

That month we had a pretty big snowstorm. It snowed the kids in for a week or so, which was fun. We baked cookies, made hot cocoa, snuggled up while watching movies and even bundled up to play in the snow. Sometimes I wonder if God helped bring that snow our way, just because he knew I needed the down time with the kids.

The excitement for chemo to end was building, but I was also feeling pretty rough. Between the fatigue and the effects of the steroids, it wasn't fun. The steroids, chemo and anxiety would cause my heart to race just out of the blue. It was so scary, and I remember crying to my oncologist with just four more treatments to go, telling him that I couldn't do anymore of it. He reassured me that I would be just fine and that we needed to finish. It would be best so we could get rid of the cancer. With lots of time in prayer with God, and trusting what my doctor said, I continued. Besides, I'm a daughter of the King, and He had great things in store for me.

I started realizing all that God was helping me through. On my lowest days I would sit on the couch, holding my bible against me, and laying my head into the couch, pretending as though I was laying in His arms. I have never felt so close to Him. It was pure peace, nothing I'd ever felt before, unless we count the day I was saved by His amazing grace. His peace poured over me in waves and it felt so real like He was right there. No matter if I wanted to cry my eyes out or praise Him, He always showed up, just like He always has.

The last week in February came and that meant it was the last chemo! We kept the kids out of school that day and took them with us. This was something to celebrate as a family. We had grown so close during my cancer diagnosis. My parents even traveled to the center to be there with us.

The kids weren't so sure when they were hooking my port up for pre-meds and chemo, they stood back in the corner of my room. Catie would watch every little thing that went on like she was a little fascinated, but Nathan didn't want any part of it. I kind of felt bad. Once we finished up, I stepped out of the room where my parents were and looked out towards the door, the nurses were lined up both sides of the hallway cheering me on! I asked the

kids if they wanted to help me
ring the bell, but with
everything going on, they
didn't know what to think. I
hugged the nurses as I inched
closer to the bell, crying my
eyes out and thanking God for
being with me every step of the
way. Ringing that bell was the
most relieving, exhilarating,
and happiest days of my life!
There is no other way to
explain it. I felt like the longest
and hardest part was over.
Now, we just waited on
surgery. Later after we left the
hospital, a few of our friends
met us for dinner to celebrate.
The very next day my friend
Robin picked me up for dinner
and I had no idea until we

arrived that she planned a surprise dinner with some church ladies and my grandma. What a sweet surprise! Lots of laughter and friendship were just what I needed to celebrate and how special of those ladies to plan this.

Because I had chemo and my immune system was lowered, I had to wait a month before I could have surgery. This was a perfect time for me to rest up and hopefully gain some energy back.

What a better way for me to rest up than to spend a weekend away with some great friends from church. Our annual Ladies Retreat fell right between chemo and the big surgery date. We usually leave on a Friday afternoon and return Sunday in time for church service. My heart craves this trip every year. After the previous six months, I really needed some good fellowship and friendship. We'll usually have a lesson the first night, stay up late and talk, then the next morning breakfast, lesson, lunch, hike, lesson, dinner, stay up late again, then breakfast on Sunday and head back towards town for church. Except that year for me there was no staying up late and the hike consisted of several breaks. I think the girls even had to bring the church van to pick me up, as I couldn't finish the walk. But oh, what a soul soothing joy it was to get away!

As the weeks and days inched closer to surgery, I was mostly excited, and just a little nervous. I had jumped one hurdle, now I just needed to get over the last one. My doctor and I agreed that as young as I was that having a bilateral mastectomy was what needed to be done, especially after having several spots on both breasts and my cancerous tumor was growing aggressively.

While waiting for surgery I tried to prepare for that down time by packaging some freezer meals and cleaning the house up some. My energy wasn't really coming back much so it was a little disappointing to be folding laundry and have to sit on the bed to rest between everything I was hanging up or folding. My husband was helping one day in particular, and he reassured me that in due time I would be back to normal and to not be discouraged. It has always been hard for me to just let things be and give up control. God taught me so much in that department and even today it's still hard, but I've come to realize more quickly in a tough season that I indeed, do need the rest, and remember that He is in control of it all.

<u>Chapter 9</u>

"She is clothed in strength and dignity,

she laughs without fear of the future."

Proverbs 31:25

I was scheduled to start surgery at seven o'clock. It was too early, and I was way too tired that morning to decide if I was nervous or not. We met my parents and left town about four thirty that morning. Surgery would last several hours but we weren't sure exactly how long. After checking in we headed upstairs to the surgical unit. I was only in the waiting room for about ten minutes or so until they called my name. I gave everyone a hug and my Dad said they would see me soon (Ok, I'm crying already over here).

I changed into a gown, made myself comfortable in the bed and waited. A few minutes later a nurse came in to prep me, started my IV and made sure my socks and surgical hat were on, then told me that my surgeon would be there soon. She also asked what my husband's name was and she would get him for me so I could see him once more before surgery. He and my parents came back for a few minutes which was nice, since I was a teensie bit nervous. I can always count on my husband to make me laugh in situations like this. They did ask me if I had any good medicine yet because my gown was on crooked and when I went to fix it, it almost flew open. Sorry, Dad!

It wasn't but a few minutes later we heard both my oncology and plastic surgeons coming up the hall toward my room, so we said our good-byes again and off they went.

Dr Partin stuck around, viewed my history in the computer, asked the nurse a ton of questions and then administered some blue radioactive dye into my breast. She explained that once back in surgery, she would cut into my armpit and remove the lymph nodes that were lit up blue, these would be the nodes that my breast drained into. I can remember laying back on my pillow afterwards as they wheeled me to the operating room. It was so bright and cold back there. They moved me from that warm bed to a more, narrow one that was freezing. I laid back on the table as they strapped me in and put a mask over my face, the nurse told me to start counting to ten, or twenty, oh I don't remember. I think I said onnnneee, and that's it.

It was a pretty extensive surgery, about seven hours long, but only felt like a quick nap to me. I remember laying in recovery, starting to come to, my mouth was so dry, and I drifted in and out of sleep. Once I was more awake and began to realize what had just took place, I looked down my gown to see how different I looked, but I was wrapped in so much bandage and a large sports bra type contraption that I couldn't see anything. The nurse realized I was awake and brought me some water to drink. About twenty minutes later she brought my family back. They tried to talk to me, but I was in and out of it. I remember thinking that I was hearing a dog barking, but my Step-Mom was trying to tell me that I indeed wasn't. She did later tell me that each time I heard a dog barking it was actually a man across recovery from me coughing, he had just had lung surgery. I feel terrible for thinking that.

I started feeling nauseas so my parents wandered to the gift shop to see if they could find me some mints. I think they came back with blow pop suckers, but it helped.

My surgery that day was seven hours long, which meant I was out of surgery early to mid-afternoon. We did hear word from my surgeon while in recovery that my lymph nodes removed showed no cancer! Praise God! The pathology report about everything else would not be back for another week.

About five hours later they finally had a room available for us. I had to stay at least one night for pain control and to be watched. I had an inkling that this would be a painful surgery but wasn't expecting how bad it really did feel. Once the good pain meds started wearing off, is when I started feeling bad. The pain was so unbearable. It was all I could do to get up to the side of the bed and stand up to get to the bathroom. Just like any hospital stay you don't get much sleep while you're there. They came in every little bit to check my vitals and close to midnight they started me on an antibiotic. About two hours later I woke up feeling flushed and my heart was racing. We buzzed for the nurse and she said I must have been having an allergic reaction, but she would have to get a doctor to approve taking me off of it and see about giving me Benadryl.

It was a little aggravating, but they finally started the Benadryl and kept me on the antibiotic the rest of the night. The next morning, they did vitals, brought breakfast and soon after that my plastic surgeon came in. With him he brought about five or six residences. A little awkward, but I understand they have to learn. Before he took a look under the bandages, he asked how I was feeling, and I told him how our night went with the antibiotic. He was pretty upset that they still had it dripping, so he had a few words with them. He then came back to check out the drains that I had, along with

the incisions that were made. I
didn't want to look so I stared
up at the ceiling. It was all too
much for me. After he wrapped
me back up, he showed us how
to empty the drains that were
coming out my sides. I really
felt like an octopus. He
explained that we needed to
log by mL how much we
emptied out at a time and the
times that we logged it. I was
also prescribed some muscle
relaxers and Tylenol for the
pain. We had been told that if I
kept up with the pain meds
around the clock then I should
do just fine. That afternoon I
was discharged, and we were
excited to get home to the kids.

Anytime throughout this journey that I had chemo and before my surgeries we would take the kids to my Grandmas or parent's house the night before and then they would take them to school the next morning. I knew that they were in great hands, but after we left them, I became so angry that the cancer was separating us. That was close to twenty times in five months that we all spent a night apart. Maybe more if we count other times when I had chemo and the side effects were so bad that they didn't need to be around to see me like that. It just wasn't fair for them.

It felt great though knowing that this big surgery was over and the last part of it was a small reconstructive surgery a few months later. The ride home was a little bumpy and any little minor bump or roughness in the road would hurt so bad, luckily, I had a "mastectomy pillow" that my Step-Mom made for me. This was nice to just lay against me whether we were in the vehicle or if I was sitting in the chair resting. Speaking of the chair, that was where I slept for the next few weeks. I could not bring myself to lay flat because of the craziest feeling that took over. Almost like an elephant was laying on my chest. I was also afraid that if I laid in the bed at night, my husband would throw his arm over me while asleep like he usually does, and that wouldn't end well.

My surgery fell less than a week before Easter, one of my favorite times of the year. I told my husband that I would be well enough to go to church that Sunday, so he took me shopping for an Easter dress. Not too much fun shopping with your husband in the first place and you know that anything you pick out now will look different because you've lost a part of your body to this awful disease. I picked out a dress though and went to church that Sunday ready to celebrate Jesus' resurrection!

It wasn't too long after my mastectomy that I was able to lift my arms above my head, dress myself and do some light housework. I did try to vacuum one day, in particular, about six weeks after surgery but was totally defeated. I had no upper body strength to push that thing across the carpet. I was slowly beginning to see a difference in my energy levels, so that was a good thing.

My results were back from surgery. We saw a radiation oncologist per my doctor because he thought I should have radiation done since there was a residual amount of tumor left that chemo did not get. She began reading some of the report and stated that she didn't think I needed it. The reason being was because my report read *"Lymph nodes clear, small residual tumor left, but showed WIDE CLEAR MARGINS"*. She looked at me and said *"Mrs. Hoover, we can't understand why, with the type of tumor that you had, which is known for branching out and not contained, that it has these very wide, clear margins?!"* I then looked at her and said, *"That was the hand of God!"*

With the mastectomy, I chose
to have reconstruction. So, at
the time of surgery once they
removed the breast tissue, they
placed tissue expanders. My
plastic surgeon began filling
the expanders just two weeks
after the mastectomy. I went
back every two weeks after for
about two months to have fills.
Once we were at the desired
size, a surgery date was set,
and they switched out the
expanders for implants. I was
also put on a maintenance drug
called Aromasin and a monthly
injection in the belly of Zoladex
for ten years. They work
together to rid my body of any
hormones, as that was what fed
my tumor. They have a few

side effects like bone loss and joint pain but help against the risk of recurrence. I also take a Calcium + Vitamin D supplement along with them.

About a week before I had the reconstructive surgery, my friend Robin texted me and broke the news that she had just found out that she had breast cancer. I remember having so many emotions roll through my body. It felt like I was hearing my diagnosis all over again. I just wanted to crawl through the phone and wrap my arms around her and be there for her! I thought, *Why?? Why does cancer have to be so cruel and invade our lives??*

It has been three years now and Robin can call herself a survivor! Her diagnosis pushed me even harder to advocate and fight. I encourage women of all ages to have regular check-ups, mammograms and just be aware of their bodies. I never thought in a million years that I would have cancer, but here I am, one in eight. I'm so very grateful to God for each new day and that I have the opportunity to tell you of how He carried me through. I just needed a little faith.

<u>Chapter 10</u>

"You have been assigned this mountain to show others it can be moved."

After coming out of a nearly one-year battle with cancer, I felt that God had placed on my heart to start writing. It was unclear at first where I should begin. So, I had an idea that maybe I should start with a simple newsletter at my church that would include a small devotional about once a month. I began writing and wrote for a few months and then stopped.

To be honest, life after cancer was not at all what I had imagined it to be. In my mind I thought everything would bounce back to normal. Well, things were far from normal. I was adjusting to the hormone blockers which brought on hot flashes, the most awful mood swings and joint pain. A combination of all of the above didn't make for a pleasant person to be around. If you don't believe me, just ask my husband. Haha!

I began keeping busy with my photography business. In fact, too busy. My family and friends would remind me to slow down, but after being down for a whole year, it was the last thing I wanted to hear.

My mind kept going back to the newsletters I wrote for the church. I felt like I had let my church family down. Struggling to keep up with work and dealing with these side effects from my medication, my head wasn't in the right place. So, I thought that I wouldn't produce anything worthy enough to read.

About two and a half years out from my last surgery I began listening to God's voice. He was telling me to slow down. My body and energy were not at all like it used to be before cancer. I mean, come on, didn't cancer teach me a lesson here?! I needed to S-L-O-W down!

I began thinking more about writing and started working on a website. Somewhere that I could blog and have a place for my photography and other creative thoughts. After starting the blog and talking about my story, I decided that maybe writing a book would be a great way to help others through their breast cancer journey and have one place to share it all at once. It's funny, back in high school I would tell my friends that I was going to write a book someday. They asked what kind of book I would write, in which I replied- *"I have no idea!"*. Well, now I have something to write about.

Again, I didn't make the time to sit down and write. I would talk about it but didn't even know where to start. I noticed though, not too long after, that God started placing people and opportunities in my path to get me on track with this idea. It was just making the time to actually start. I would put the kids to bed at night and pick up a notepad and pen, but nothing was flowing. I became very impatient and thought maybe it wasn't supposed to be. I wanted it so bad, but I just didn't know where to begin writing.

Earlier this summer I started thinking about how I could expand my photography business and build that studio/she shed I've always dreamt of. I found a spot behind our house that would be perfect! It was right inside the woods and was just plain magical. One day in particular I was researching small business loans and looking on Pinterest for building plans. When my husband came home from work that evening, I presented him with all of these ideas and information that I had researched. We measured off a few places and you could tell he wasn't too sure about it. If you know anything about us, then you know I'm a fly by the seat of your pants kind of gal and he's very cautious and takes forever to make a decision. Well, after measuring and talking some about it, he walked on up the hill and I leaned against the tree, still dreaming about it, I started talking to God. I presented my plans and poured out my excitement to Him! After reminiscing I walked up the hill towards my husband. We picked up a few sticks, put them in a burn pile and then started to head back to the house. I, of course, started walking straight down the hill, while he walked across. I was also wearing flip-flops. Do we know where this story is heading? Just about a half a second after he said, *"walk across the hill"* and I said, *"I know what I'm doing"*, I started sliding straight down. My left foot kept going, and my root foot stayed behind. My toes curled back, and I heard a loud *"POP!"*. I had not actually fallen, but after that, I quickly sat myself down. The ground was a little damp and full of twigs, *ouch!* My husband ran over to me and I wasn't sure if I would cry or scream, nothing was coming out. I'm not sure if he first asked if I was alright or if he was lecturing me on hiking in flip-flops. It might have been the other way around, not sure, I was in a lot of pain! Our sweet pup, Sadie ran straight up the hill to see about me. She laid down and started sniffing my foot, sensing that something had happened. My son, Nathan wasn't too far behind her. They tried to walk me across the hill, but I could only rely on one leg and like I said, the ground was

very damp. We stood there
brainstorming on a way to
bring me down off the hill.
Then my husband had an ah-ha
moment and said *"Nathan, stay
here with your Mom. I'll go get
the tractor and we can use that!"*.
After what seemed like an
eternity, but in reality, was
only three minutes, he came up
the hill on the John Deere
tractor with the bucket on the
front. I'm sure it was all a
funny sight to see me riding in
the tractor bucket, but I could
have cared less. We arrived at
the hospital and the x-ray
confirmed it was broken in two
spots. I had a cast placed a few
days later and was told it
would be about a six week

downtime. I just couldn't believe it. Why had this happened? It sure was going to be a long summer sitting at home. I cried for the first week, a lot! Mostly because I couldn't do anything for myself and had to rely on everyone else. Then one morning, something hit me. I thought to myself- *"I need to write this book!" Maybe, just maybe, this happened so I would slow down and finish what God had laid on my heart!"*

Boy, I hope I'm not the only one that's stubborn. Sometimes I'm a slow learner when it comes to God's calling. I saw a quote not too long ago by Morgan Harper Nichols that says, *"She does not know what the future holds, but she is still grateful for slow and steady growth"*. So true, but especially on the slow part. I like to think too that maybe God didn't think I was quite ready to write yet. All too often I'll make decisions or assume that I know what He wants me to do. I need to remember, it's always in His timing!

It's not been too bad of a summer. My foot is healing up nicely, I spent time focusing on my children, this book and it all worked out for God's glory! When He has a plan, nothing will stand in the way of it. I am so humbled and honored that

He asked me to be the storyteller of His amazing grace and love.

Being diagnosed with cancer will change you, most of the time for the better. I quickly learned what was most important in this life. It's certainly not the cars we drive, big, fancy or perfect houses, brand name clothes, or chasing after things we don't need. When you're faced with death, you only think about those that you love. You think about how much that you loved. You think about memories that you've made. You hope with everything in you that you'll have a chance to make more of

those memories. For tomorrow
is not promised. Live for the
day you are in and live it well!

If you..........

Are afraid:

"For the battle is not yours, but God's."

2 Chronicles 20:15

Need strength:

God is in the

midst of her;

she shall not

be moved.

God will help her when morning dawns.

Psalm 46:5

Need healing:

"Take heart daughter, your faith has made you well." Matthew 9:22

Are weak:

"She is clothed in strength and dignity, she laughs without fear of the future." Proverbs 31:25

Need peace:

"Be still and know that I am God."

Psalm 46:10

Need faith:

So do not

*fear, for I am
with you; Do
not be
dismayed, for
I am your
God. I will
strengthen
you and help
you; I will
uphold you
with my
righteous
right hand.
Isaiah 41:10*

Are feeling stressed/tired:

Rest in the Lord, and wait patiently for Him.

Psalm 37:7

"Come to Me, all who are weary and heavily burdened and I will give you rest."

Matthew 11:28

Acknowledgements

James, thank you for pushing me around this summer in that wheelchair with my broken foot, because I saw the fear in your eyes when I was learning to walk with the crutches. I think it was best for everyone's safety. More than anything, thank you for supporting me in all that I do. I love you.

Nathan, thank you for being completely honest with me when I asked you if I should add anything more to the book and in all seriousness you replied with- *"Can you put my YouTube channel in there*

somewhere?" Haha! I love you,
son.

Catie, my beautiful, sweet and
spunky daughter, I pray that
you never have to hear the
words *Breast Cancer* in your
future. Thank you for being my
best friend through this
journey. I love you, pretty girl.

Dad and Mom (Denise), thank
you for praying and believing
in everything that I do,
especially this book!

Grandma and Grandpa,
you've asked every week when
the book would be finished.
Well, here it is! Thank you for
your endless support, I love
you both!

Michelle, from the time I decided to write this book you were behind me one-hundred and one percent. Thank you for your kind words and endless support!

Robin, where do I even start? Thank you for being a listening ear and a shoulder to cry on. God had a plan five years ago when our paths crossed. Little did we know all that we would go through together! Thank you for your encouragement and support as I put my story into writing.

Mike, without you and your guidance, I would not know where to begin with putting this story out there. Thank you for answering my many, many questions!

Wayne, thank you for your patience in creating the cover and helping with the layouts. I couldn't have done it without you.

Elaine, not many people would take work on vacation with them! Thank you for going out of your way to be the best editor and friend a girl could ask for. Thank you for the grammar checks and your ideas for the book. I truly appreciate it!

Casey, my beautiful photographer friend. I explained my vision for the cover of the book and you delivered! Thank you for the wonderful photos and your friendship.

Other thanks goes out to: My Christian sisters at CFC, my many friends with whom I shared thoughts about this book with, Dinah's Boutique, and Three Little Buds (Joanna).